Yeast Infection Guide

A Natural Candida Cure to Boost your Immune System and Achieve Optimal Health with a Complete Candida Cleanse and Candida Diet

LILY PHILLIPS

TABLE OF CONTENTS

INTRODUCTION

I want to thank you and congratulate you for purchasing the book, *"**Yeast Infection Guide**: A Natural Candida Cure to Boost Your Immune System and Achieve Optimal Health with a Complete Candida Cleanse and Candida Diet."*

This book contains proven steps and strategies on how to:

- Recognize the signs and symptoms of yeast infection

- Distinguish yeast infection from other types of infections through a reliable diagnosis and consultation with your physician

- Identify the cause of your yeast infection that will prompt you to seek the best solution

- Discover that you have several treatment options aside from the typical drug-based prescription of your physician

- Benefit from a complete Candida cleanse and diet plan that will get rid of the cause of your yeast infection naturally

- Heal your immune system from the damage brought by Candida albicans – the root of yeast infection

- Rebuild a stronger immune system that will serve as your impenetrable defense against Candida yeast

You will also find from this book several sample recipes that will help in cleansing your body and boosting your immune system to gain your freedom from yeast infection.

Thanks again for purchasing this book, I hope you enjoy it! Please take some time to stop by and LIKE our Facebook page:

https://www.facebook.com/joypublishing

With gratitude,

LILY PHILLIPS

Chapter 1
WHAT YOU NEED TO KNOW ABOUT CANDIDA YEAST INFECTION

One of the first things you have to do to solve the problem is to get to understand it better. This way, you can make better decisions that will give you long-lasting freedom from Candida yeast infection.

What the Problem Is?

Yeast infection or Candidiasis is a type of infection resulting from a multiplication of fungus, specifically yeast, in the body. The most common type of yeast that affects both men and women is Candida Albicans, hence the alter-nickname. Candidiasis is also the most common among yeast infections.

According the WebMD, Candida Albicans, also called monilia, is a fungus that typically lives in the human body in negligible amounts. You can usually find this fungus on your skin, mouth, rectum, and often in the vaginal area. However, Candida Albicans may also travel inside your body through your blood and reach your intestines, heart, and throat.

In negligible amounts, you do not have to worry about the presence of this fungus. But, when the fungus starts to multiply, there is a greater risk of infection. If the overgrowth is unmanaged or uncontrolled, the infection may become worse. It is also important that you prevent the fungus to enter your bloodstream.

Causes of Candida Yeast Infection

Frequently, Candida yeast infections just happen, with no seeming reason. While the exact cause is difficult to pinpoint, health experts concur that any changes in the environment of the body can trigger an overgrowth of the fungus and the infection follows thereafter.

The common reasons for body environmental change are the following:

- Having a weak immune system is a common cause of yeast infection. To those who have compromised immune systems, the infection can affect the entire body and may be life threatening without proper treatment.

  Furthermore, statistics show that 15% of persons with a compromised immune system acquire systemic illnesses with Candida yeast as the cause.

- Use of drug-based medicines, especially antibiotics and steroids. This is because synthetic medicines (such as antibiotics) also kill the good bacteria that prevent fungus (like Candida Albicans) to grow out of control.

- In women, aside from synthetic medicines, other reasons for the change are the following: pregnancy, pills for birth control, diabetes, menstruation especially the menopausal stages. In men, failure to undergo circumcision is a risk factor.

- Use of medical devices that have to be inserted or embedded into the skin is another risk factor. Examples of these devices are catheters as well as intravenous ports. Persons who use unsterilized needles are also at risk.

Signs and Symptoms

Watch out for the following, as they may signal you that you have Candida yeast infection:

Vaginal Yeast Infection

- Thick, white discharge which resembles cottage cheese

- Vaginal itching and irritation which can range from mild to severe

- Burning sensation during urination

- Pain when having sexual intercourse

- Labia is sore, red, and sometimes swollen

Yeast Infection in Men

- Pain during urination

- Penile skin irritation

- Redness, dryness, and flakiness of the tip of the penis or the penile area under the foreskin(for uncircumcised men)

Oral Candidiasis

- Formation of thick patches that are white in color atop a red base located in the mouth, usually on the tongue and palate

- Pain in difficulty in eating your food due to the presence of the patches inside your mouth

How to Diagnose Candida Yeast Infection?

Consulting with your physician is the best way to determine that what you have is yeast infection. This is because the symptoms may sometimes resemble that of the symptoms of vaginal bacterial infection.

In diagnosing healthy patients, usually physicians only need to look at the affected area (e.g. vagina, penis) and can readily tell the infection. In most instances, they will recommend gynecological diagnostic tests, such as vaginal swabbing, to rule out other infections.

If the physician suspects that the yeast infection may have entered the bloodstream, your doctor may recommend a more invasive diagnostic test for confirmation.

Do You Need Medical Treatment?

It is prudent to consult with your physician to diagnose the infection. Treating the infection, however, does not require medical intervention right away. In most instances, natural remedies and cures are enough to control the infection, prevent the risk factors, and get rid of the cause of your condition.

You may need medical treatment if and when:

- The symptoms continue to persist despite natural treatment

- Recurring infections that may already be a symptom of a more serious health condition, such as AIDS or leukemia

- The presence of blood in your discharge

- Skin rashes or lesions that do not heal within two weeks

- The infection is accompanied by chills, fever, nausea, and vomiting, and the discharge comes with abdominal or stomach pain

- The infection results with loss of appetite for food and reluctance to drink fluids

Chapter 2
THE CANDIDA DIET

Are you aware that your body is capable of healing itself without the use of synthetic medicines? Health conditions, such as Candida yeast infection, are easily treatable and preventable through eating the right diet.

> "The food you eat can be either the safest and most powerful form of medicine or the slowest form of poison."-Ann Wigmore

As the father of medicine once said, "*Let food be thy medicine and let medicine be thy food*" (Hippocrates); thus, the food that you eat determines the kind of health that you enjoy.

That said, your diet is perhaps the key solution that will enable you to get rid of the cause of your yeast infection. Eliminating the cause will prevent Candida yeast from recurring and wreaking havoc to your good health. It matters that you choose your food wisely, as it can either be your tool to get well from your condition or it can worsen the infection.

Why You Can Benefit from the Diet?

A Candida diet plan is one of your fundamental tools to stop and control yeast infection. This is because like human beings, the fungus that cause the infection, Candida albicans, need food in order to grow, survive, and multiply. You need to stop the cycle and the best way to do that is to deny these fungi their source of life and nourishment, and that is food.

The main source of nourishment and food for Candida is also the food that brings the most health risks to human beings. This food is sugar. You may find several variations of the Candida diet plan, but these variations have a common denominator, and that is to eliminate or limit your sugar consumption to treat the infection. If you starve the Candida albicans, they will die. The rest of them, realizing that they can hardly survive in a sugar-starved environment, will voluntarily go away from your body.

The Many Forms of Sugar

Sugar is not just the sugar that you put in your food or beverage to sweeten them. It can take various forms, such as the following:

- Lactose that you will normally find in dairy products such as milk.

- Fructose that you can find naturally from fruits and starchy vegetables.

- High fructose corn syrup is an artificial sweetener that is considered as the most dangerous type of fructose.

- Glucose is your blood sugar. Like fructose, you can also find glucose from starchy fruits and vegetables.

- Sugar substitutes such as saccharin, corn starch, galactose, dextrose, and more. One tip: if a word ends in "-ose", it is most likely to refer to sugar.

Besides sugar, Candida yeast also loves carbohydrates, especially food that contains high amounts of carbohydrate and gluten grains. Examples of these food items are the following: pasta, white breads, baked goods, potatoes, cereals, and pizza.

The common goal of Candida diet plans is to get rid of the cause of the yeast infection. The best plan will also target to strengthen your immune system, your body's primary weapon and shield against all types of infections. This way, you will benefit from long-term results that will enable you to enjoy your infection-free health for a long, long time, if not permanently.

The best diet plan does not only clear your body of Candida yeast but it will also flush out toxic substances and wastes that may have been lingering in your body for so long. After the removal of these harmful substances from your body, you will feel lighter, better, and will enjoy your improved overall health condition. Clearing of toxins will also allow you to lose your excess weight.

Treating your yeast infection with an anti-Candida diet will not only clear your body of the fungus, but will also promote your overall health.

Food to Avoid to Treat and Prevent Candida Infection

Following is the list of food to avoid in treating and preventing the infection:

FOOD TYPE

Sugar

Sugar, sugar substitutes or artificial sweeteners, syrups, honey, chocolate, molasses, soft drinks, diet colas as they contain aspartame that can weaken your immune system and increase your vulnerability to yeast infection.

Grains and Glutens

Wheat, barley malt, elbow macaroni and other pasta, cakes, bread and bread crumbs, pastries, cereals, pre-cooked meat, rice, corn and byproducts, such as popcorn

Fruits

Fresh, canned, dries, and fruit juices contain natural sugars. Lemon is allowed. For preventive purposes, eat fruits in moderation, as fruits are good for your health.

Vegetables

Potatoes, sweet potatoes, beets, carrots, peas, yams. Once your yeast infection is cleared, reintroduce these veggies into your diet one at a time as these vegetables have high nutrient density.

Meat

Canned meat products, all pork meat and products, processed meat, cured meat, packed meat, smoked meat

Fish

Almost all fish meat except salmon (the wild variety) and sardines, all shellfish

Dairy products

Milk, buttermilk, cheese, and whey. You may consume butter, kefir, and yogurt (preferably unflavored).

Alcohol

All types of alcoholic beverages as they do not only contain high sugar, but they also weaken your immune system.

Other Types of Beverages

Energy drinks, soft drinks (regular and diet), coffee, fruit juices, tea (black, green)

Oils

Corn, peanut, canola, soy

Vinegar

All except for apple cider vinegar

Condiments

Soy sauce, ketchup, mayonnaise, tomato paste, spaghetti sauce, relish, mustard

Nuts

Cashews, pistachio, peanuts

Beans & Mushrooms

Tofu, soy cheese, soy milk, legumes, mushrooms

Additives/Preservatives

Citric acid, any odd-sounding ingredients in the food label can disturb your natural microflora, triggering yeast infection

Food You Should Eat More Often

Here is a list of foods that you should eat more often to treat and prevent the occurrence of a Candida yeast infection:

FOOD TYPE

Non-starchy vegetables

Asparagus, broccoli, Brussels sprouts, cabbage, celery, cucumber, raw garlic, kale, onions, spinach, tomatoes

Yogurt (Live cultures)

Probiotic yogurt, kefir. The live cultures will repopulate your gut with good bacteria that will allow you to regain control of Candida yeast to treat and prevent infections.

Gluten-free grains

Quinoa, oat bran. Their rich fiber content will cleanse your digestive system that is necessary in eliminating the Candida fungi

Nuts and seeds

Almond, hazelnut, pecan, walnut, sunflower seeds, flaxseed, coconut meat

Meat

Lamb, beef, turkey, and chicken (choose fresh, organic, and preferably lean cut)

Fish

Wild salmon, anchovies, sardines, and herring

Oils

Virgin coconut oil, olive oil, flaxseed oil, sesame oil, and red palm oil

Beverages

Tea (ginger, cinnamon, peppermint, licorice) as it contains anti-Candida yeast properties

Sugar substitutes

Stevia, xylitol

Herbs and spices

Black pepper, basil, cinnamon, cloves, ginger, garlic, oregano, rosemary, thyme. These herbs and spices enhance the flavor of your meals where recipe ingredients may be limited due to a strict Candida diet.

Condiments, seasoning

Sea salt, lemon juice, apple cider vinegar

Anti-Candida Diet Recipes

Here are some recipes that you can use as guide to prepare your meals when you are on a Candida diet:

Sample Breakfast Recipe

Kale Egg Breakfast

Ingredients

- 2 pcs eggs
- 2 large-sized Kale leaves with the stems
- Virgin coconut oil
- A pinch of sea salt

Procedure

1. In your blender or food processor, combine the eggs, kale leaves with stems, and sea salt.

2. Blend the ingredients until they arrive at your desired texture or consistency.

3. Set your stove at medium heat. Pour a few drops of virgin coconut oil in your pan for heating.

4. Pour your blended kale egg mixture in the pan. As soon as the eggs start to cook, scramble.

5. When the mixture has reached your desired level of doneness, turn off your stove.

6. Let the kale egg mixture cool a bit before serving.

Sample Lunch Recipe

Chicken Curry

Ingredients

- About one (1) pound of chicken cut into small servings
- One onion, sliced
- 3 pcs tomatoes, chopped
- 2 cloves of garlic, crushed
- One teaspoon of minced ginger
- A can of coconut milk
- One pc of red bell pepper (remove the seeds)
- Half a teaspoon of cayenne pepper
- Half a teaspoon of turmeric powder
- Half a teaspoon of curry powder
- One teaspoon of virgin coconut oil

Procedure

1. In a pan, pour your coconut oil and sauté the onion, tomatoes, garlic, ginger, and bell pepper.

2. Add the chicken. Cook for about 5-10 minutes.

3. Add the rest of the ingredients. Adjust the heat to low. Cook for about 30 minutes or until the chicken reaches your desired doneness.

4. Let the dish cool a bit before serving.

Sample Dinner Recipe

Broccoli with Beef

Ingredients

- About one pound of beef cut into small pieces or strips
- One pound of broccoli florets
- 2 cloves of garlic, minced
- 1 white onion
- Half a teaspoon of cayenne pepper
- Half a teaspoon of butter
- Sea salt and black pepper to taste
- Virgin coconut oil for sautéing

Procedure

1. In a pan, pour a few drops of virgin coconut oil. Add the butter, and then the onion and garlic. Sauté.

2. Add the beef strips and cook for about 3-5 minutes in high heat.

3. Adjust the heat settings to medium-low. Add the broccoli florets and cayenne pepper along with salt and pepper to taste. Cook for about 2-3 minutes.

4. Let the dish cool a bit and then serve.

Sample Snack Recipe

Yummy Avocado

Ingredients

- 1 large avocado
- 1 clove garlic, grated
- ½ white onion
- Fresh lemon juice
- Cilantro
- Sea salt to taste (optional)

Procedure

1. Chop your ingredients.

2. Combine them in a mixing bowl.

3. Garnish with cilantro.

4. Serve.

Tips and Techniques to Get the Most Benefit from Your Diet

Preparing Your Meals

- Before you go to the grocery store, create your meal plan for the week. List all the ingredients that you need, and make sure that the list does not contain ingredients that are in the list of foods to avoid while following a Candida diet.

- Print the list and bring it with you to the grocery store. It is also important that you know how to read food labels. Sugar can come in various names such as the following: fructose, dextrose, maltose, fruit juice concentrates, invert sugar, glucose, and a hundred other aliases.

- Choose non-starchy vegetables that are also low in carbohydrates and glycemic index, and high in nutrient density. You may want to use the *low-glycemic vegetable list by Dr. Oz.* Here are a few examples:

  ❖ Artichokes
  ❖ Asparagus
  ❖ Brussels sprouts
  ❖ Cucumber
  ❖ Okra
  ❖ Onions
  ❖ Peppers
  ❖ Radish
  ❖ Cabbage

  Note that some vegetables in the list (e.g. beans) are food items to avoid. Just refer to the table provided earlier and cross the items out of Dr. Oz's list.

- Limiting your carbohydrate intake will benefit you, speeding up your healing and recovery process from Candida yeast infection. Include food ingredients that regulate your blood sugar levels. For instance, green leafy vegetables along with avocado make an ideal combination in combating the Candida yeast.

- As much as you can, skip any food that is baked or has dairy content. While on a Candida diet, you should stay away from food containing yeast and dairy products, such as milk and cheese. f you have to include cheese as an ingredient, choose lactose-free cheese.

- Increase the amount and number of herbs and spices in your recipes. They will make up for your limited ingredients, as herbs and spices are effective in enhancing the flavors and taste of your meals.

Chapter 3
YOUR COMPLETE CANDIDA CLEANSE

Consulting your physician is necessary and important to get an accurate diagnosis of your infection. As mentioned earlier, many of the symptoms of Candida yeast infection are similar to symptoms of bacterial infections. The diagnosis will be able to tell the difference and confirm your infection as coming from Candida yeast.

When it comes to treatment, however, know that you have several options. Most physicians will readily recommend anti-fungal drug-based medicines because it is what they are trained to do. While these medicines bring immediate relief of the symptoms, they rarely address the cause of the problem.

It is wise to start your treatment with natural remedies and go for a complete Candida cleanse. These remedies work well with your body to fight the infection and bring more long-lasting results. The reason is that natural remedies work to fight the cause of the yeast infection, which you can attribute to the uncontrolled growth of Candida albicans in your body because of changes in your body's environment.

Why Perform a Complete Candida Cleanse

In getting rid of the cause of your Candida yeast infection, it is crucial that you prepare your body to get the most benefit from the treatment. One of the first things that you need to do is to cleanse your body, specifically your colon as this is where toxins, wastes, and the Candida yeasts usually linger.

Uncontrolled growth of Candida albicans in your digestive tract is what causes yeast infection. This growth is primarily due to changes in your body as discussed in chapter 1 of this book. It becomes easy for the albicans to grow and thrive in your intestinal tract when your body is loaded with toxins and wastes that destroy and overpower your good bacteria, specifically Acidophilus Lactobacilli.

Steps in Doing a Complete Candida Cleanse

Preparing For the Cleansing Diet

It is crucial that you have the right mindset in battling the yeast infection. Note that the Candida diet can be restrictive and there are several food ingredients that you will need to avoid. This is because the goal of the diet is to starve the Candida yeast until they die and give up inhabiting your body.

The thing is the nourishment they need to survive is also the food ingredients that may be the most difficult to give up for human beings. If you find yourself in such a situation, just think that eating the food that you need to avoid will only make your nemesis, the Candida albicans, stronger with their continued growth and reproduction.

Denying them their food for survival will kill them and drive the rest to seek refuge elsewhere. Hence, feeding them can only lengthen your treatment period and worsen your symptoms while starving these albicans will speed up your healing and will free you from the symptoms for good as you get rid of the cause of your yeast infection.

The Tools That You Need

Just like when you have to do real-life battles requiring that you have weapons and shields, the same is true when combating yeast infection. You need tools to win the battles and eventually the war against Candida albicans. These are the following:

- A body environment free of toxins and wastes

- A stronger immune system

- A diet that will starve the albicans and force them to retreat or die

3 Stages of Cleanse

Therefore, in doing a complete Candida cleanse, you will have to pass three (3) basic stages:

1. *Cleansing Phase* – this is where you get rid of toxic substances in your body to make sure that your digestive tract is clean and free from obstructions.

2. *Candida Dieting Phase* – this stage is where you starve the albicans to death and prevent entry to Candida yeast wanting to populate your body. This is easier to accomplish when you start with a clean and optimal digestive system.

3. *Rebuilding of your Immune System* – this stage is what will sustain the results that you achieve from the first two

stages. This is also where reintroduction of food in your diet happens.

For instance, you can reintroduce food items that you have skipped during the cleansing and dieting phase, such as fruits, with a stronger immune system. You just have to see to it that the food you reintroduce is beneficial to your overall health. Discard unhealthy food permanently and completely.

Cleansing Your Body

The cleansing stage lasts for about a week or less. The actual duration of your cleansing depends on the condition of your health and your weight. If you can allot a week to focus on doing the cleansing, the better it is to achieve faster results or shorten the duration of this phase.

In the detoxification stage, it is best to limit your food to vegetables, especially the green leafy variety, and avoid the rest of the food items even if they fall under the allowed list in the Candida diet plan. Vegetable consumption will prevent you from deprivation and hunger and they can also help in cleansing your intestinal tract as most vegetables are also natural detoxifiers.

Here is a list of 10 vegetables that can detoxify your body:

1. Asparagus

2. Bok Choy

3. Broccoli

4. Celery

5. Cucumber

6. Dandelion greens

7. Kale

8. Lettuce

9. Spinach

10. Swiss Chard

Start your detoxification diet by drinking one (1) glass of warm water before consuming your first meal in the morning. The water will perk up and prompt your kidney to do its job well.

You will also need the following as your tools for detoxification:

- Lemon water

- Detox beverage

Sample Detox Drink Recipes

Below are simple recipes in creating lemon water and another detox beverage:

LEMON-INFUSED WATER

Ingredients

- 2 to 3 slices of fresh lemon
- A quart of ice and water

Procedure

1. Immerse the fresh lemon slices in water and ice.

2. You may drink it right away or refrigerate it then drink it later.

LEMON-GINGER DETOX

Ingredients

- 1 -2 teaspoons of fresh lemon juice
- Fresh ginger (thumb-sized or one square inch)
- Two cups of water

Procedure

1. Peel the outside skin of the ginger.
2. Grate the ginger.
3. Boil the water.
4. Add the grated ginger into the boiling water and continue to boil for about 10 more minutes.
5. Strain the boiled gingered water and let it cool until you can tolerate the heat level to drink.
6. Add the lemon juice to enhance the flavor and strengthen the detox power of the drink.

Fiber for Cleansing

Consuming the following fiber will also help in cleansing your digestive system:

- *Psyllium Husks* – is one of the excellent sources of water-soluble fiber. It expands with water and the powder transforms to a soft and sticky substance. The substance will cleanse your colon and improve the consistency of your stool for easy passage. It will also attract the toxins and fungi, pull them from your colon lining, and flush them out of your body along with other wastes.

- *Aloe Vera* – promotes the general health of your digestive system. It is rich in enzymes that break sugar and starches from food and at the same time stimulating the growth of good bacteria in your body. Aloe encourages quick passing of stool reducing the transmit time of food particles. This, in turn, prevents yeasts from forming.

- *Chia Seeds* – are rich sources of dietary fiber to flush out Candida yeast from your body. When you consume the seeds, they scrape your intestinal wall to remove lingering wastes, toxins, and Candida yeast from the lining and allow your body to excrete them. These seeds also help boost your immune system to prevent the reformation of Candida yeast in your body.

Chapter 4
BOOSTING YOUR IMMUNE SYSTEM

Your immune system plays a critical role in your battles and war against Candida yeast infection. A weak and compromised immune system is a great opportunity for Candida albicans to invade your body successfully. A strong immune system will drive away these albicans and deny them entry into your body.

Interaction between the Immune System and Candida

You know that your immune system is your body's natural defense to fight and defend against Candida yeast. The enemy knows this too well; hence, Candida albicans see to it that they attack your immune system first to weaken it and thereafter invade your body.

In view of this, you need to do two things: (1) repair the damage that the Candida albicans have caused to your immune system; and (2) rebuild a stronger immune system that will deny and prevent entry to these albicans for good.

Repairing the Damage of Candida

Cleansing your body and following a strict Candida diet will repair the damage to your immune system brought by the Candida yeast infection. To heal your immune system:

- It is necessary that you restore the good balance of bacteria in your body. Your good bacteria should overpower your bad bacteria to keep your body safe from infections. It also keeps the Candida albicans under control.

  Thus, including probiotics in your diet is crucial. Probiotics promote the growth of good bacteria in your body and will restore the healthy balance that your immune system needs in order to heal and recover from the damage.

  Examples of good bacteria are Lactobacillus Acidophilus and Bifidobacterium. You will find these naturally occurring in certain foods such as yogurt and other fermented food, and there are also readily available supplements.

  If you choose to take probiotic supplements, the best thing to do is to choose them carefully for their quality. Some supplements are really made from high quality ingredients that they are able to accomplish what they claim, while other supplements fail to deliver results because of substandard quality of their ingredients.

- Minimize the stress on your immune system. You can do these by avoiding food that feed the albicans and at the same time taking vitamins and minerals that will de-stress your immune system. If you believe that you are not getting sufficient vitamins and minerals from your diet, you can benefit from taking a vitamin-and-mineral supplement, as advised by the Harvard Medical School.

Rebuilding the Immune System

You should not stop with the repair of your immune system. Once you have successfully driven away the Candida albicans and have repaired, healed, and recovered the good health condition of your immune system, the next thing you need to focus on is to rebuild your immune system to make it stronger.

A stronger immune system will allow you to enjoy all the benefits that you have gained from cleansing your body and from following the Candida diet. As your immune system blocks all possible entry of the Candida fungi, you may start to reintroduce healthy food items that you have avoided during the detoxifying and Candida dieting phases.

Healthy Diet

Following a healthy diet is one of the best methods to boost your immune system. What you eat directly affects your immune system and can dictate the condition of your health. Your immune system needs nourishment to maintain its excellent health, and you can provide this nourishment with the right choices of food.

See to it that your body is receiving the daily recommended nutrient and energy intake. If you are overweight, you will need to lose your excess weight and maintain your recommended weight thereafter. Choose food that can deliver the following micronutrients to boost your immunity against infections including Candida yeast:

- Vitamin A

- Vitamin B6

- Vitamin B2

- Vitamin D

- Vitamin C

- Vitamin E

- Selenium

- Zinc

- Folic Acid

- Iron

- Copper

Herbs to Boost Immunity

Herbs are also beneficial in boosting your immune system. Thus, it is advisable to include them in your healthy diet regimen. In choosing herbs, consider your body's unique composition and dietary needs. Make sure that the herbs you choose will bring no adverse reactions to your body.

Some of the best herbs that boost the immune system are the following:

- Echinacea – is considered as a stimulator for better immunity responses. You just have to use it sparingly or conservatively and to make sure that you are not allergic to its components.

- Garlic – is a popular natural herbal remedy that has anti-fungal, anti-microbial, anti-bacterial, and anti-parasitic properties. It is also easy to benefit from garlic as most recipes require it as an ingredient.

- Ginseng – can stimulate the optimal functions of the immune system. Several studies have already established and confirmed its ability as an immune booster and further studies are continuing to explore the full potentials of this herb.

Healthy Lifestyle

It is also important that you switch to a healthy lifestyle to sustain the benefits you get from following a healthy diet. Here are some of the things to do to make the switch:

- Increase your physical activity such as walking. You may also want to start a simple exercise regimen that you can easily integrate in your daily routine.

- Get enough sleep and relaxation. Sleep is the condition where you allow your body to recover from stress and restore the optimal functions of your body systems. Relaxing your body and mind frees you from stress.

- Improve your interpersonal relationships. Humans are basically social beings. Building a solid support system and nurturing close friendships have positive effects on your health condition and immune system.

CONCLUSION

I hope this book was able to help you to:

- Understand Candida yeast infection better. Understanding your problem will enable you to make better choices in treating and preventing the infection.

- Create your own anti-Candida diet plan using the information presented in this book as your guide or reference. Each body is unique, and the diet that may work for one may not have the same results or effects for another.

- Recognize the importance of having a clean digestive system in eliminating the cause of your problem, which is the overgrowth of Candida albicans.

- Repair and rebuild your immune system to prevent the recurrence of yeast infection and to promote your overall optimal health condition.

The next step is to maintain your consultation and coordination with your health practitioner. The content of this book is not intended to replace the findings, recommendations, or advise from your physician. You can use the content to discuss your options with your physician and to make prudent choices and decisions.

Finally, if you enjoyed this book, please take the time to share your thoughts and post a positive review on Amazon. It'd be greatly appreciated!

In addition, please remember to check out our Facebook page in order to find other resources and upcoming promotions:

https://www.facebook.com/joypublishing

With sincere thanks,

LILY PHILLIPS

ONE LAST THING...

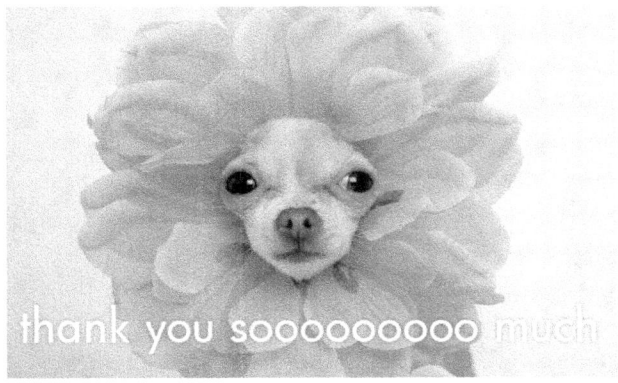

If you believe that this book is worth sharing, would you please take the time to let others know how it affected your life? If it turns out to make a difference in the lives of others, they will be forever grateful to you, as will I.